TOMMY THE ZOMBIE

Written By: Willie H. Freeman III
Illustrated By: Kimberly Anne J. Dy Buncio

Incubator Press, LLC
incubatorpress.com

In a tiny little town
called "Edison Place"
Pouts an angry little boy
very red in the face.

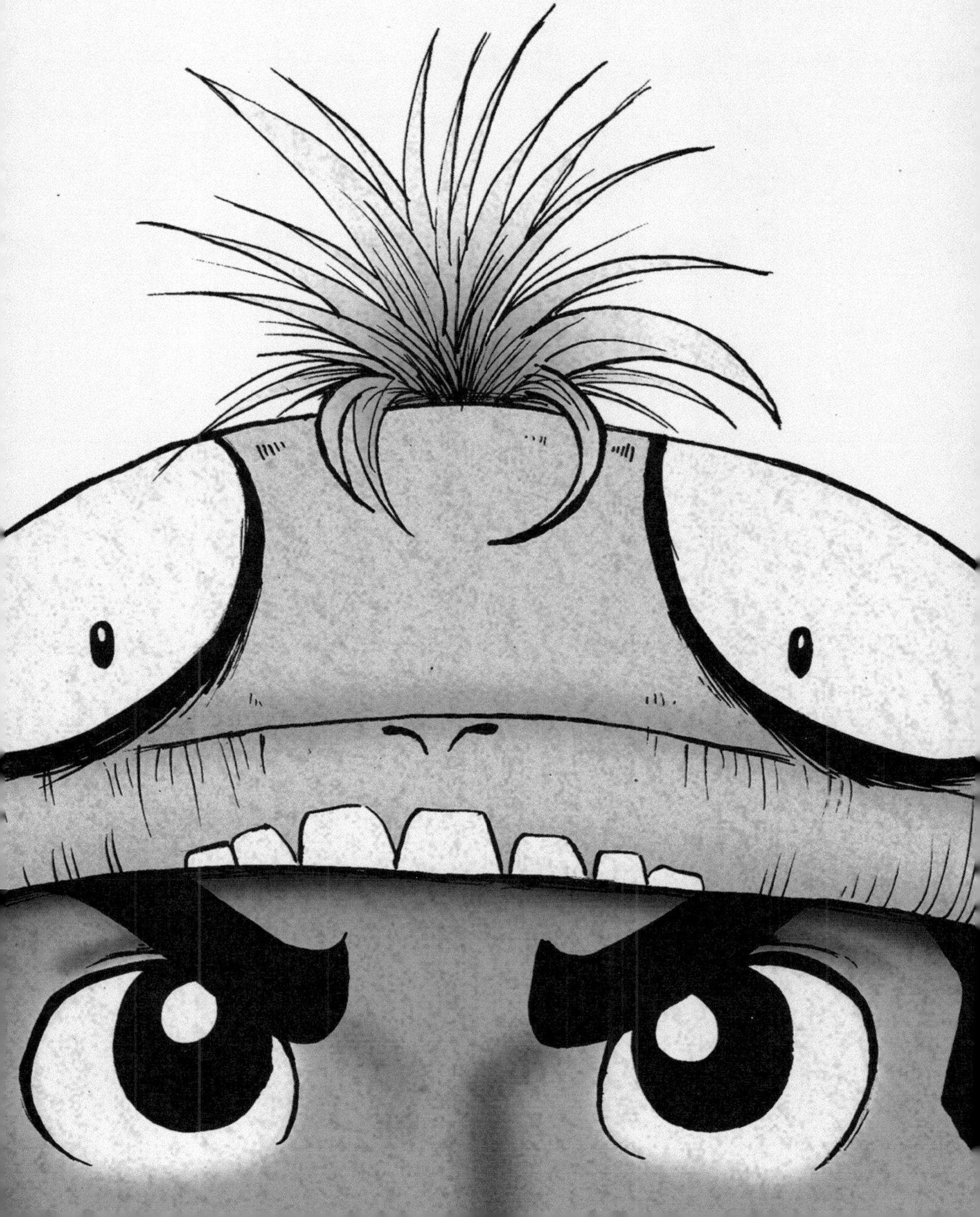

Ever since Halloween
his daddy and mommy
Have been living in fear
of a dinnertime zombie.

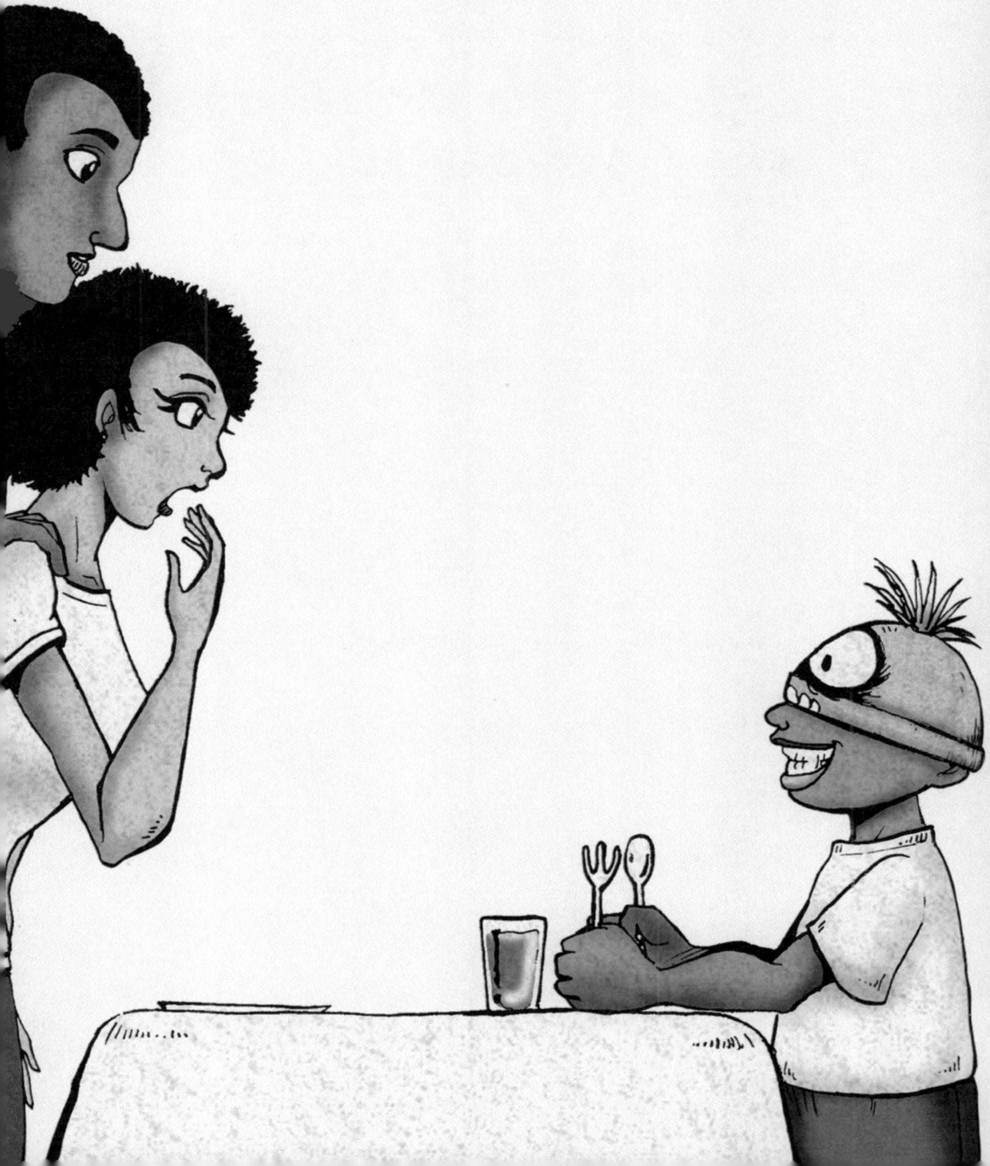

The boy's name is Tommy
and each night he strains
To escape the dinner table
where vegetables reign.

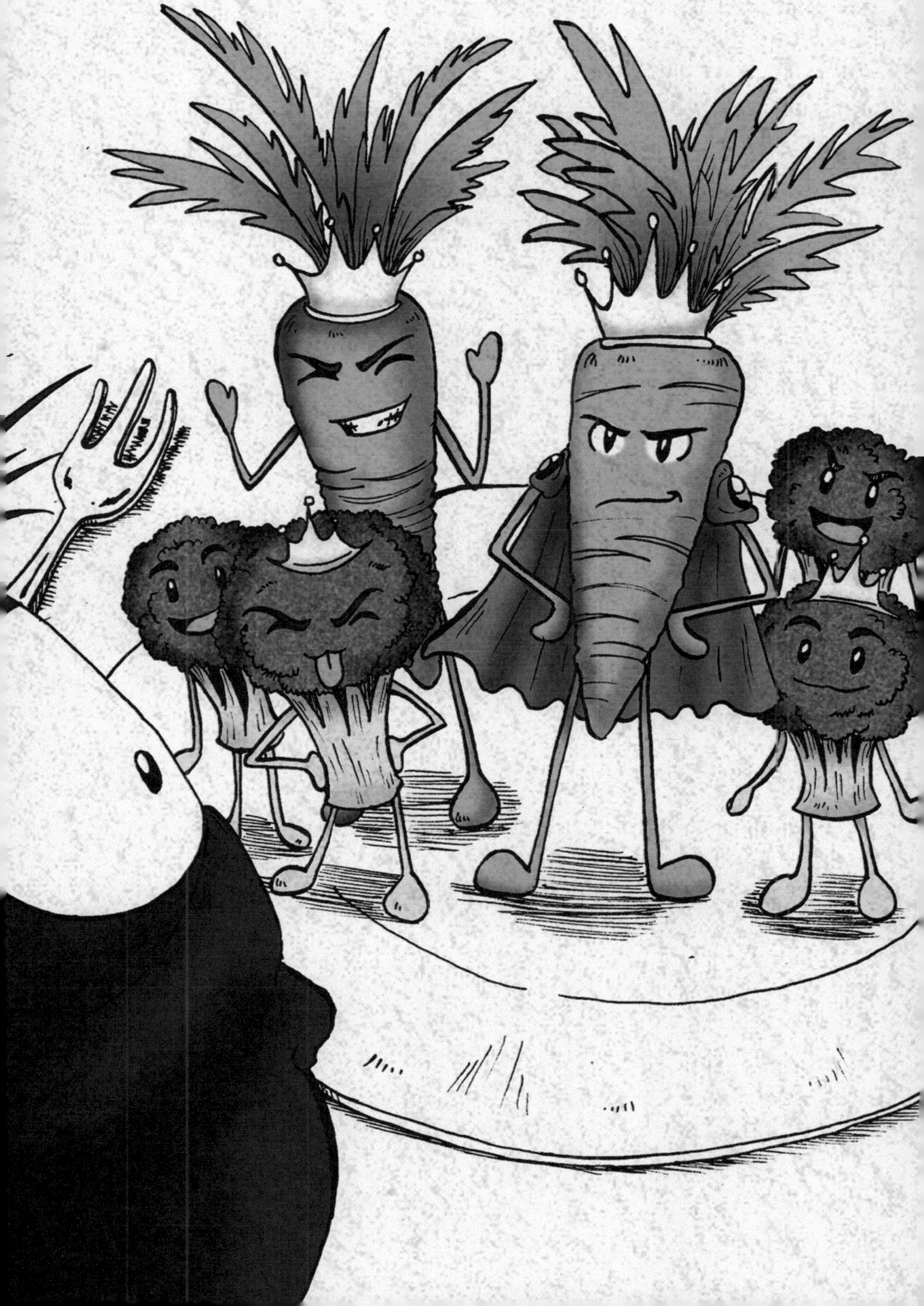

He stares and he moans,
he shuffles and groans.
He falls limp to the floor
like he's lost all his bones.

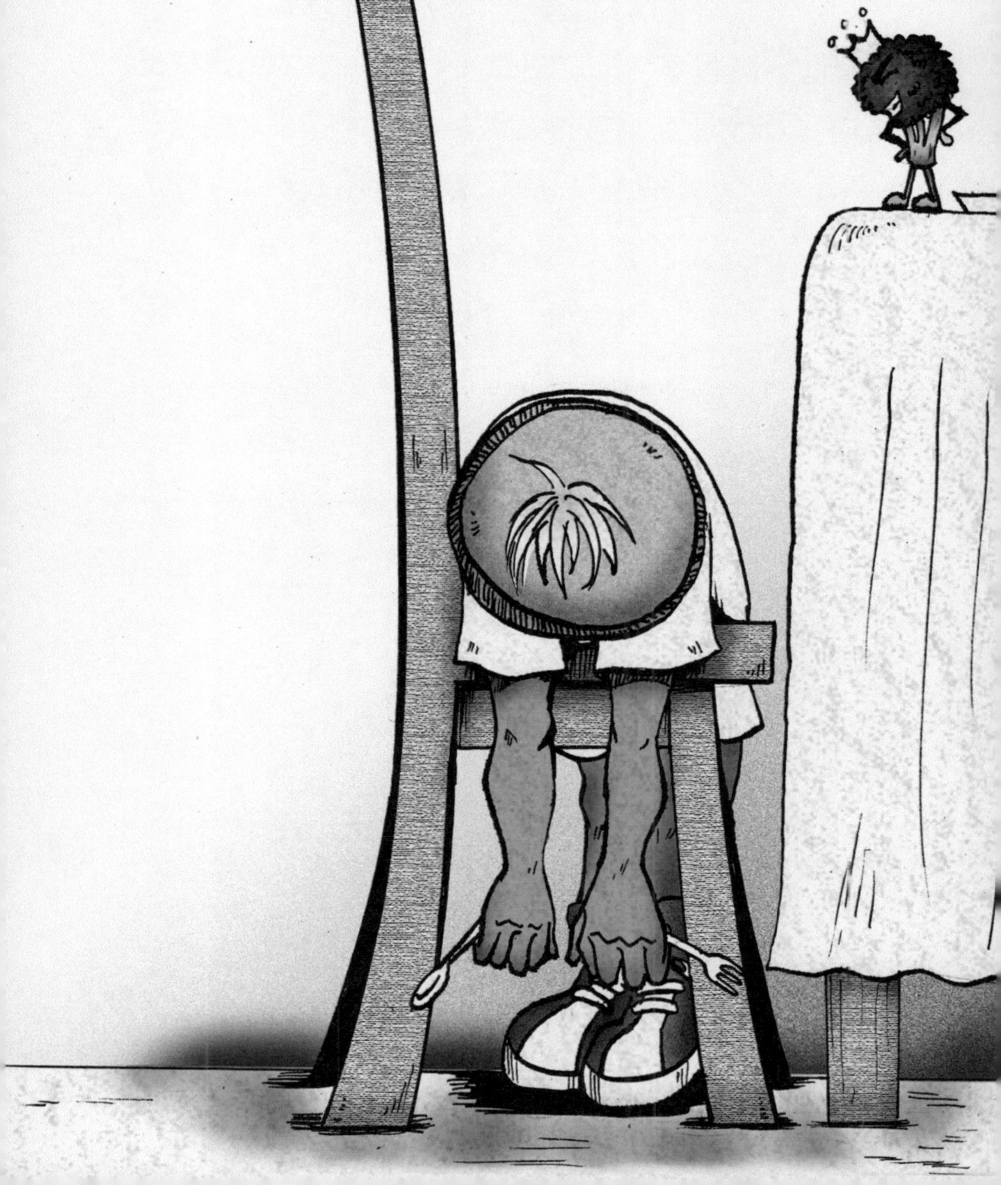

There he remains
until his parents take pains
To put him back in his chair
to start over again.

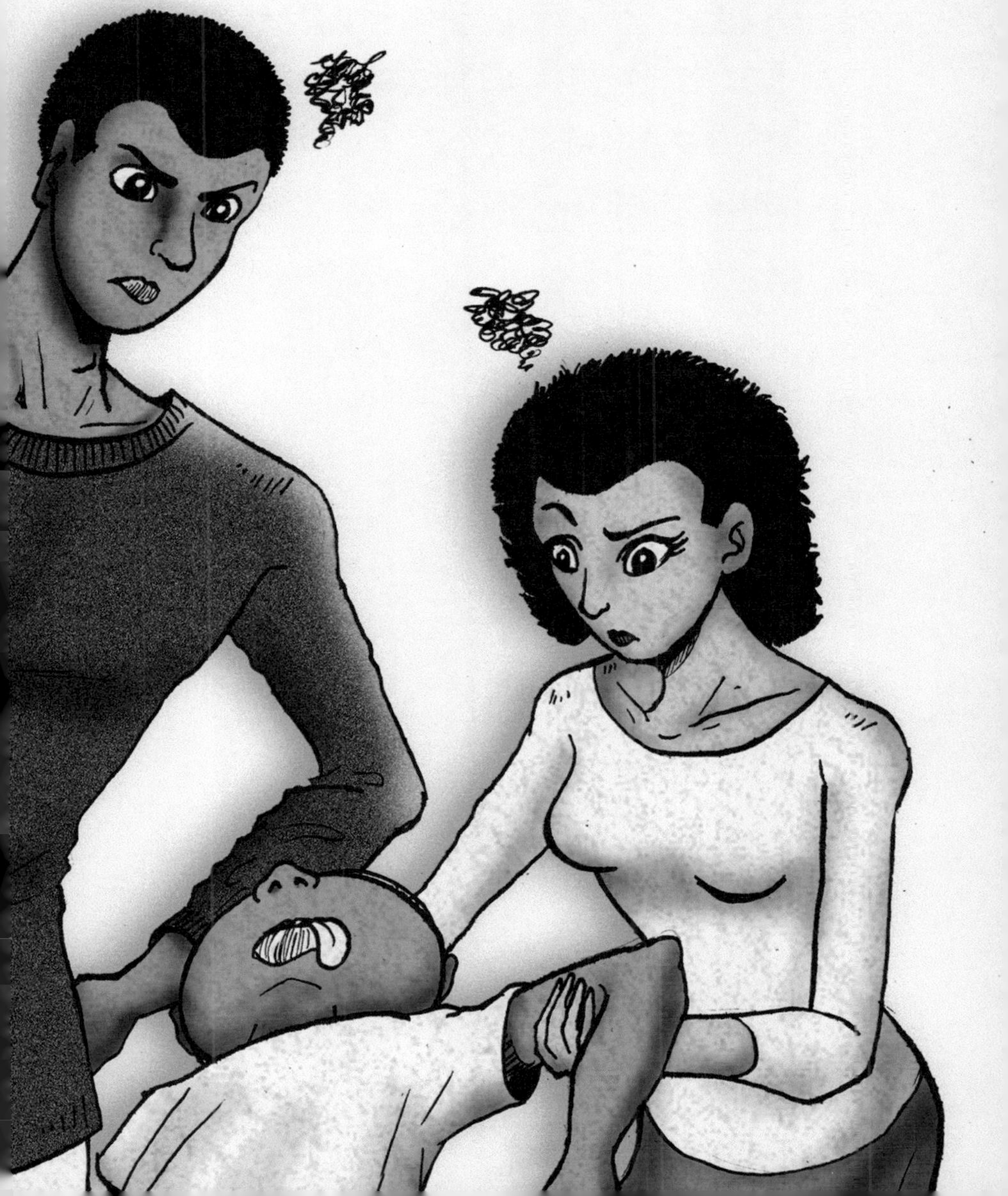

This nightly apocalypse
lasted till Christmas
As Tommy the Zombie
had worried them senseless.

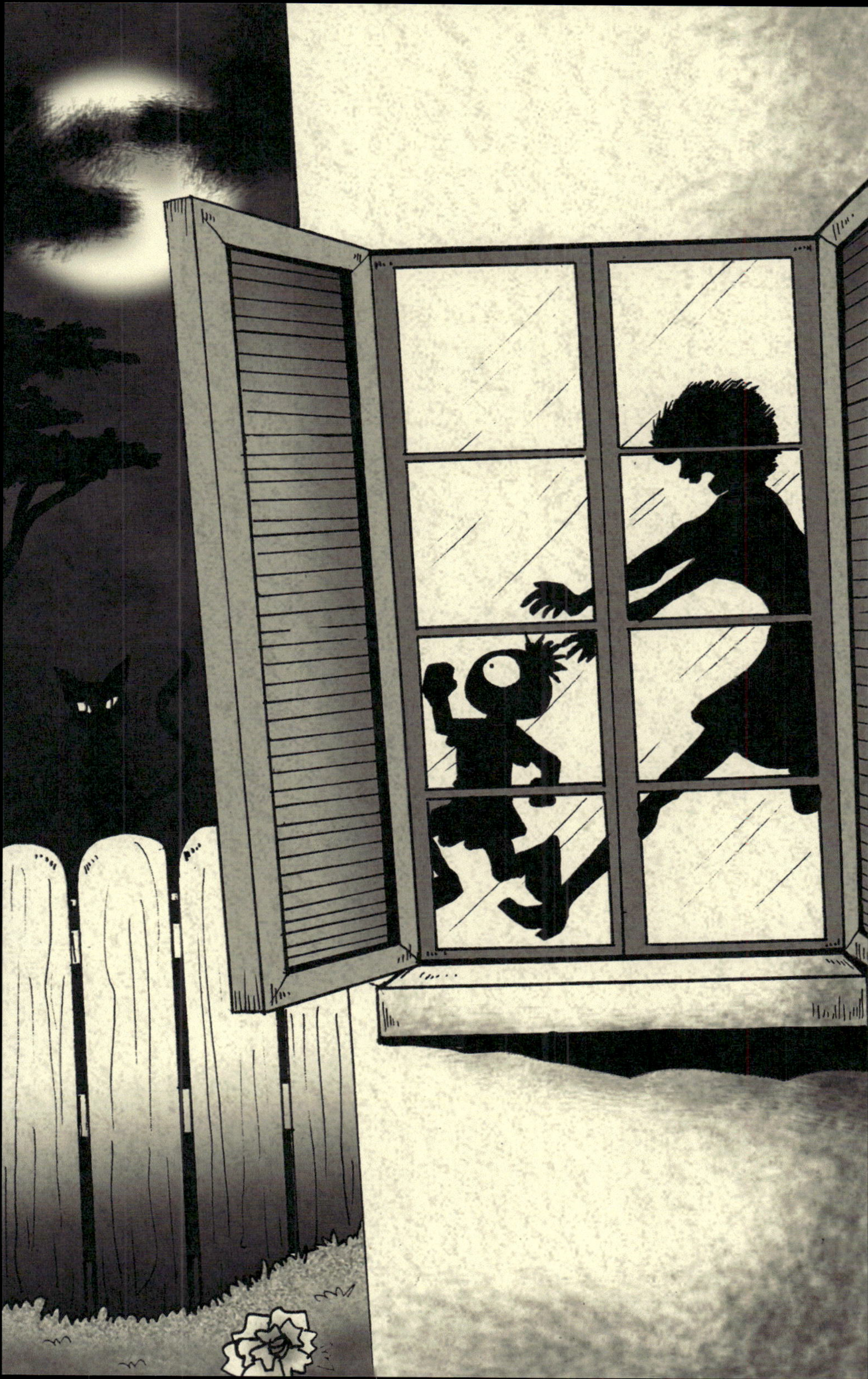

So Daddy and Mommy
decided their gifts must
Be more than just presents
and toys and fun treats
So Mommy asked Daddy,
"What do zombies eat?"

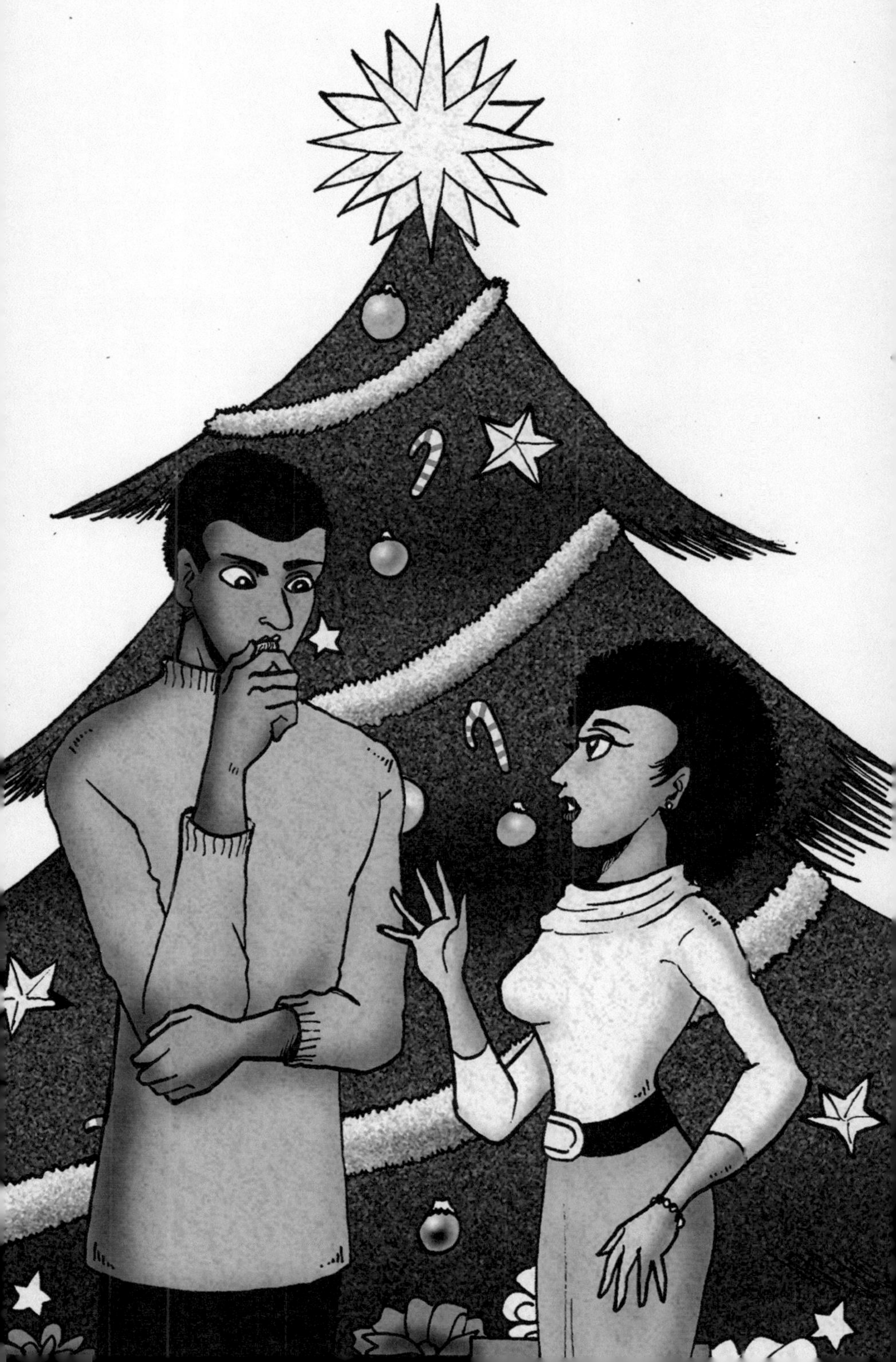

So Christmas day came
and as Mommy had asked,
Daddy gave Tommy
a new zombie mask,
some toys and a scrapbook
that came with 3 tasks.

"To be a great zombie,
first you must pass
the Zombie School test
by training for one year."
Tommy said nothing,
but grinned ear-to-ear.

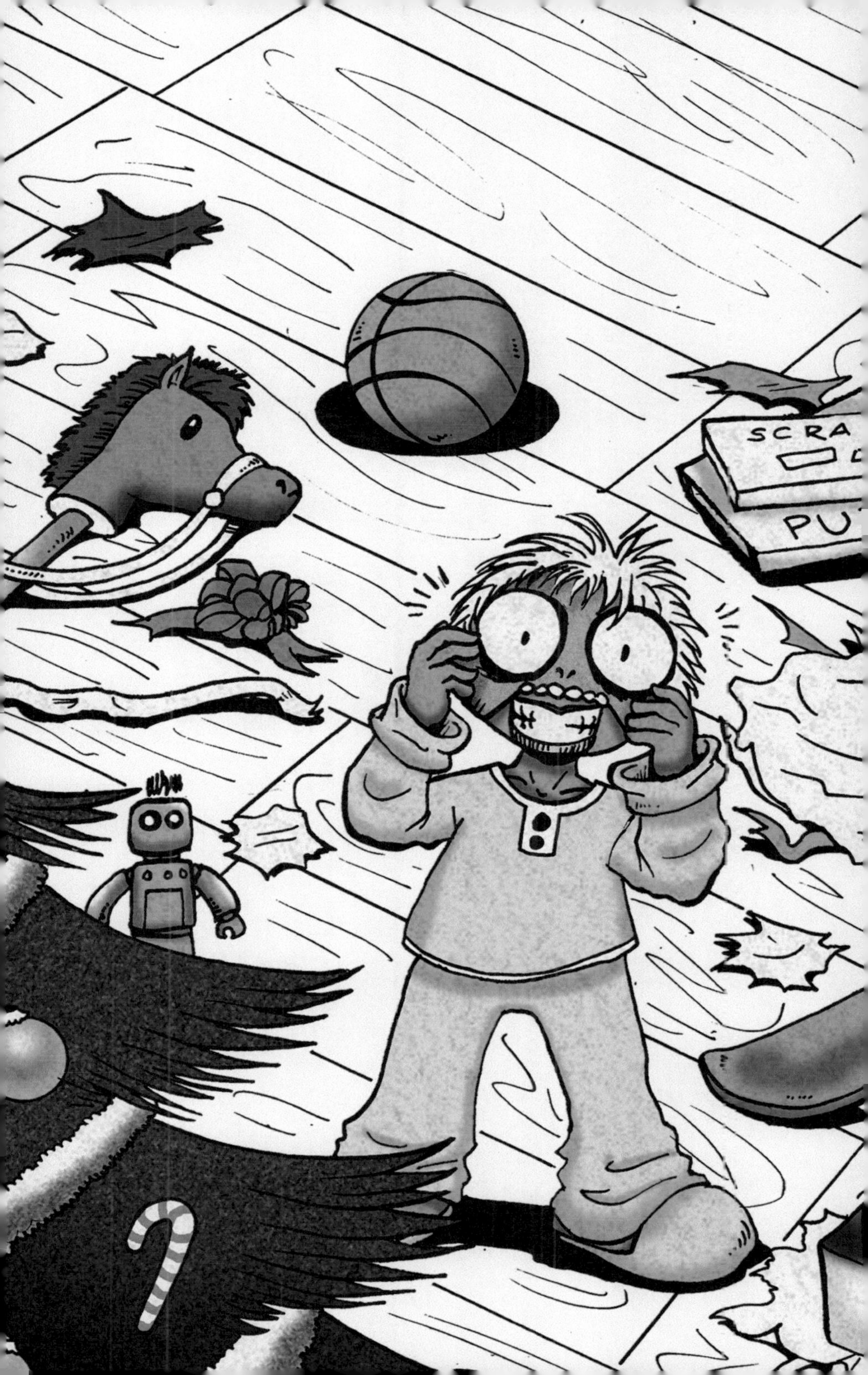
SCRA
PU

Mommy spoke next:
"Prepare for your training.
Three tasks every night
and leave none remaining.
For zombies may groan,
but there'll be no complaining."
"Are you up to this, soldier?"
his Daddy asked proudly.
"Sir, yes sir!"
roared the zombie loudly.

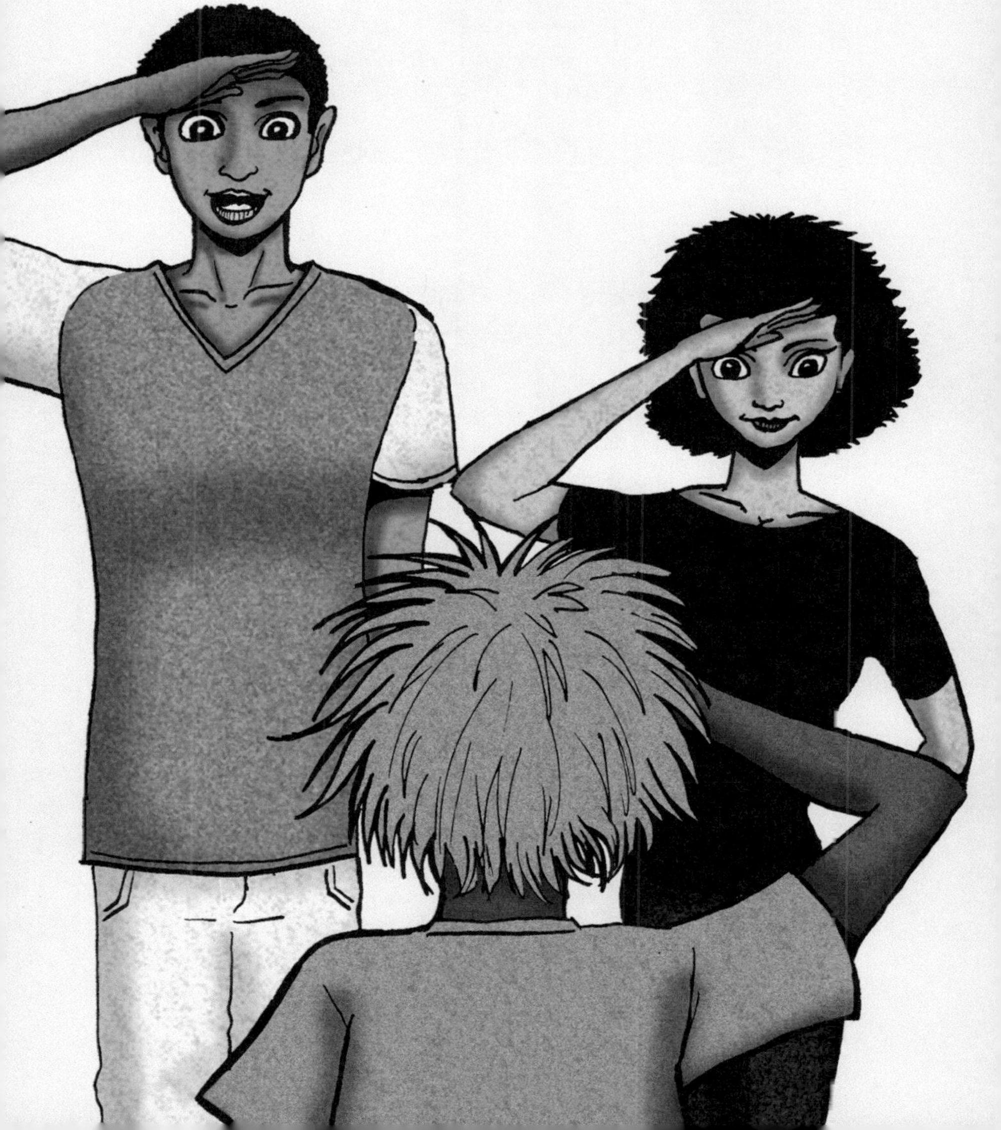

"Number one," spoke Daddy.
"A strong zombie is effective.
When they feed, they are not picky;
they are far from selective."

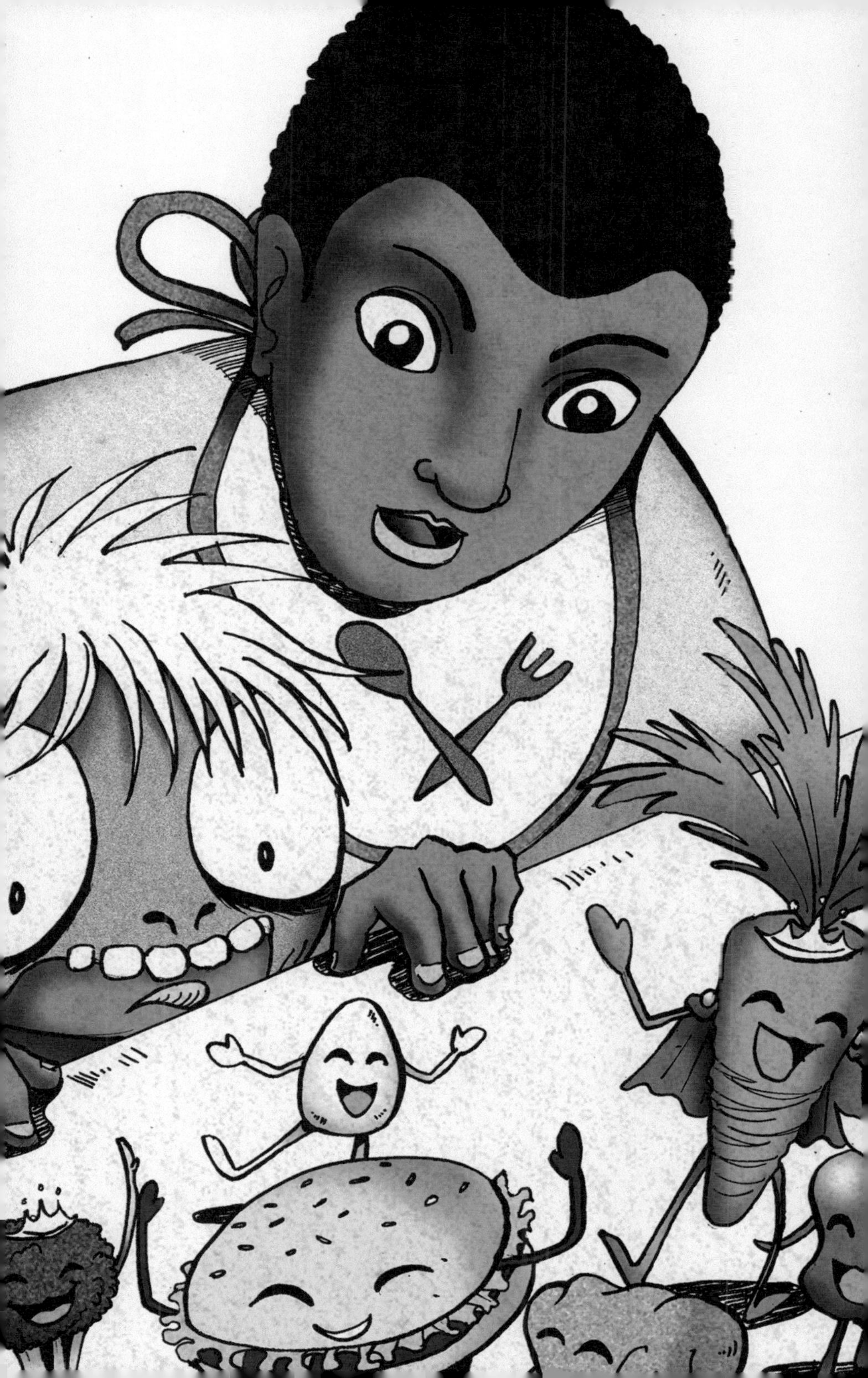

Then Mommy said softly,
"Here's number two:
Our strength is in numbers,
you'll feed when we do."

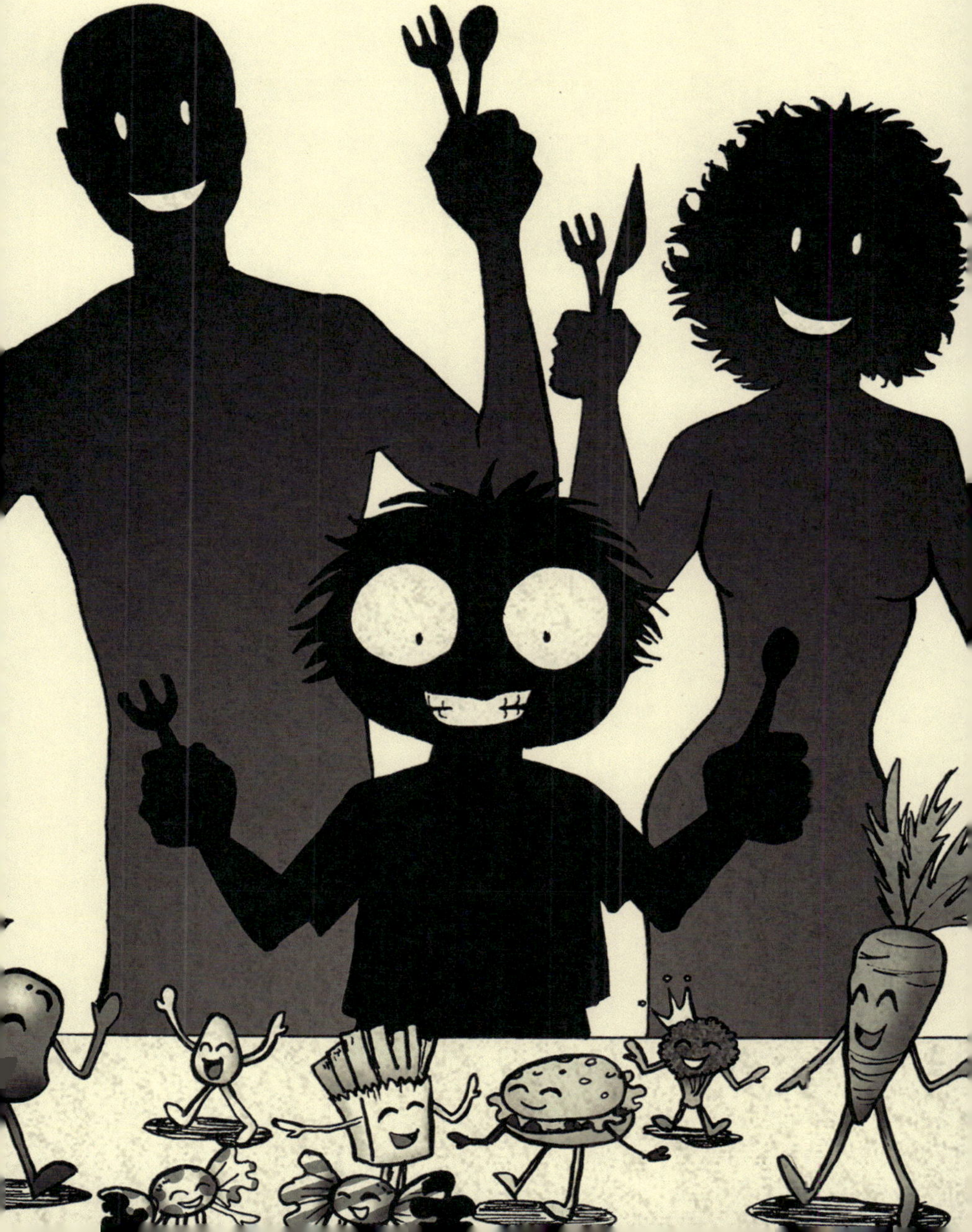

"Number three is most vital,
to a young undead fiend.
You are what you eat,
and all zombies are green."

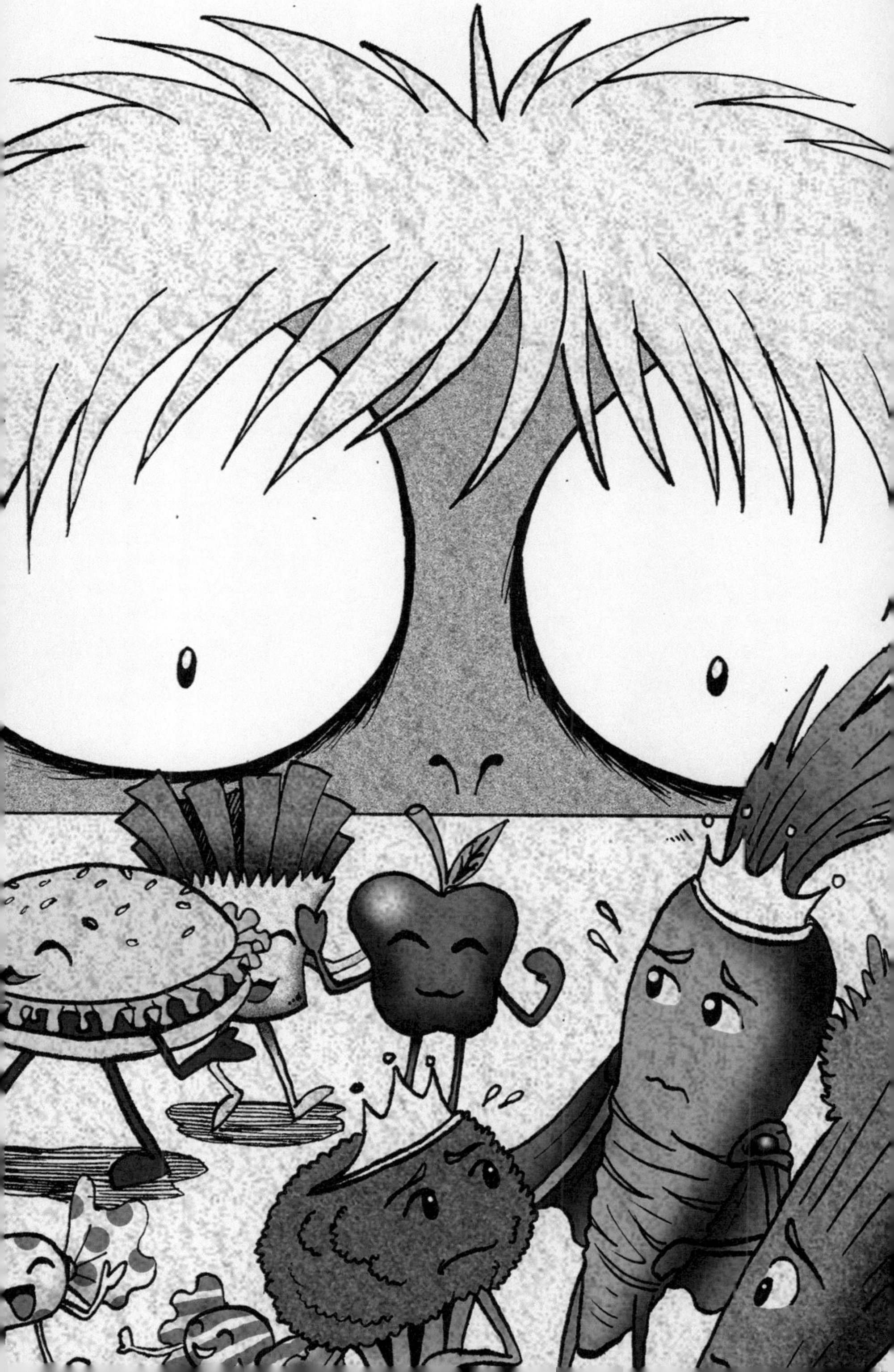

So each night for a year,
as dinner was served
in stalked a young zombie,
almost unobserved.

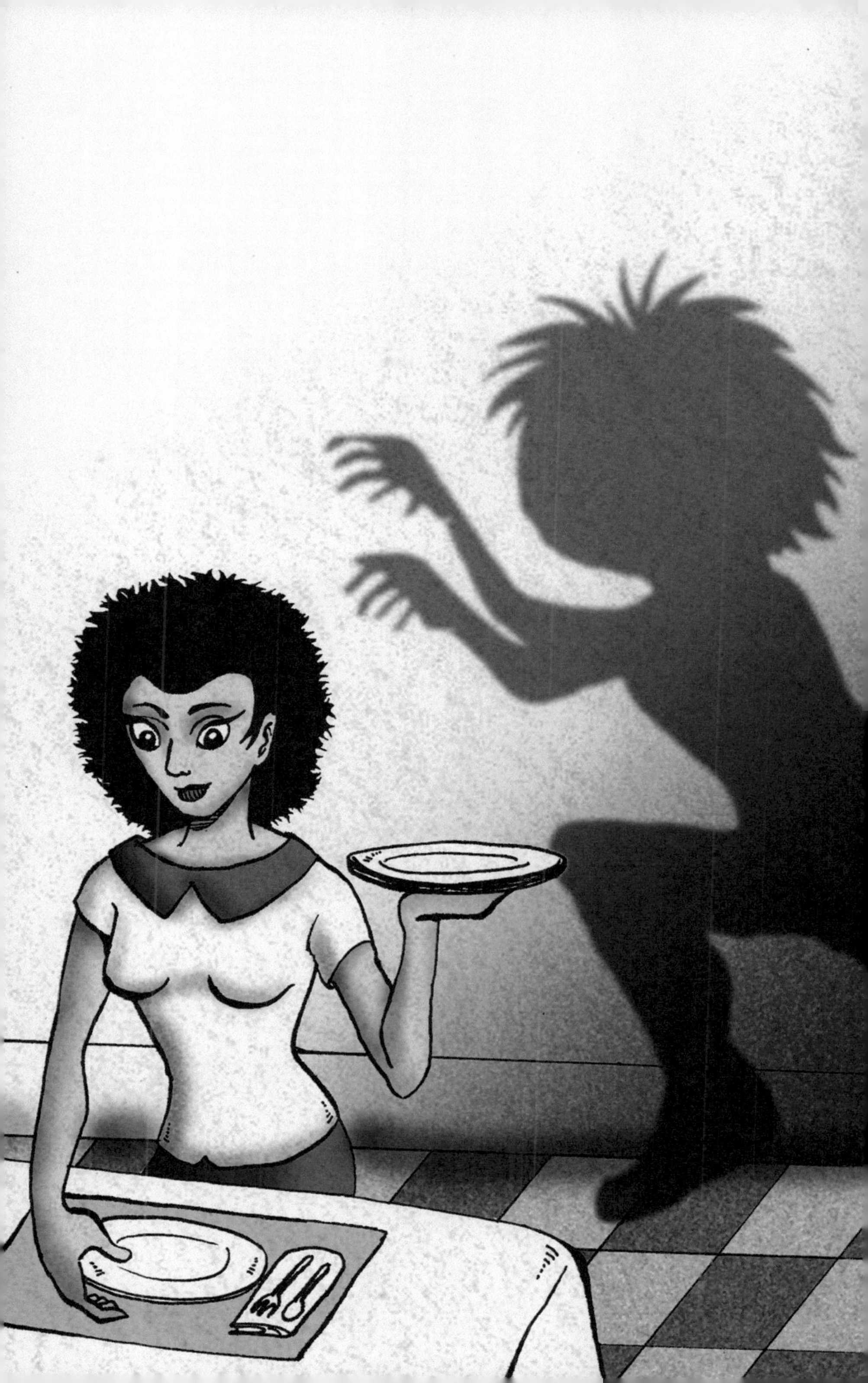

He groaned from the shadows,
he staggered and strained
toward the bright dinner table,
where vegetables reigned.

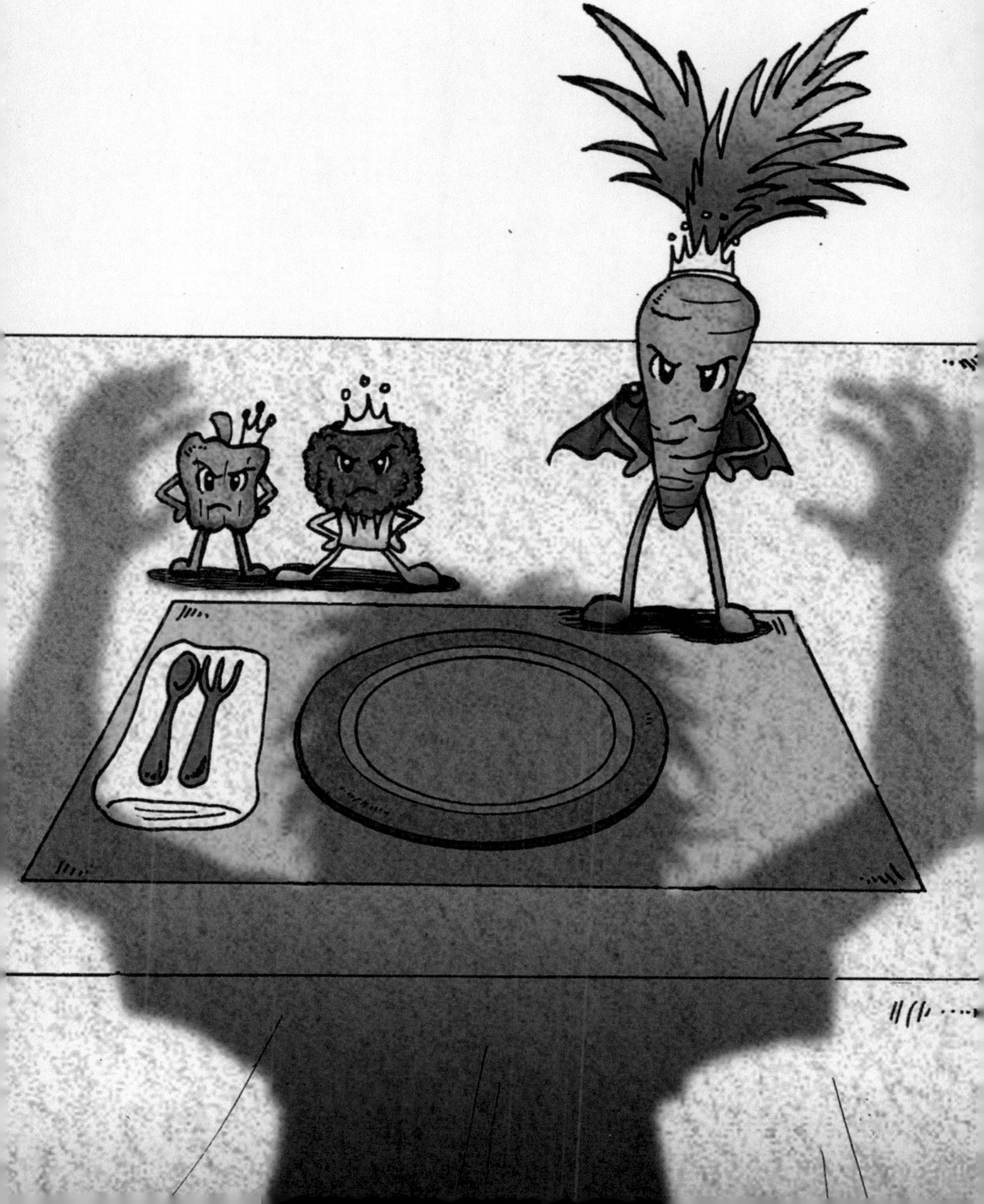

He ate everything else.
Only green stuff remained.
He remembered his promise
not to complain.

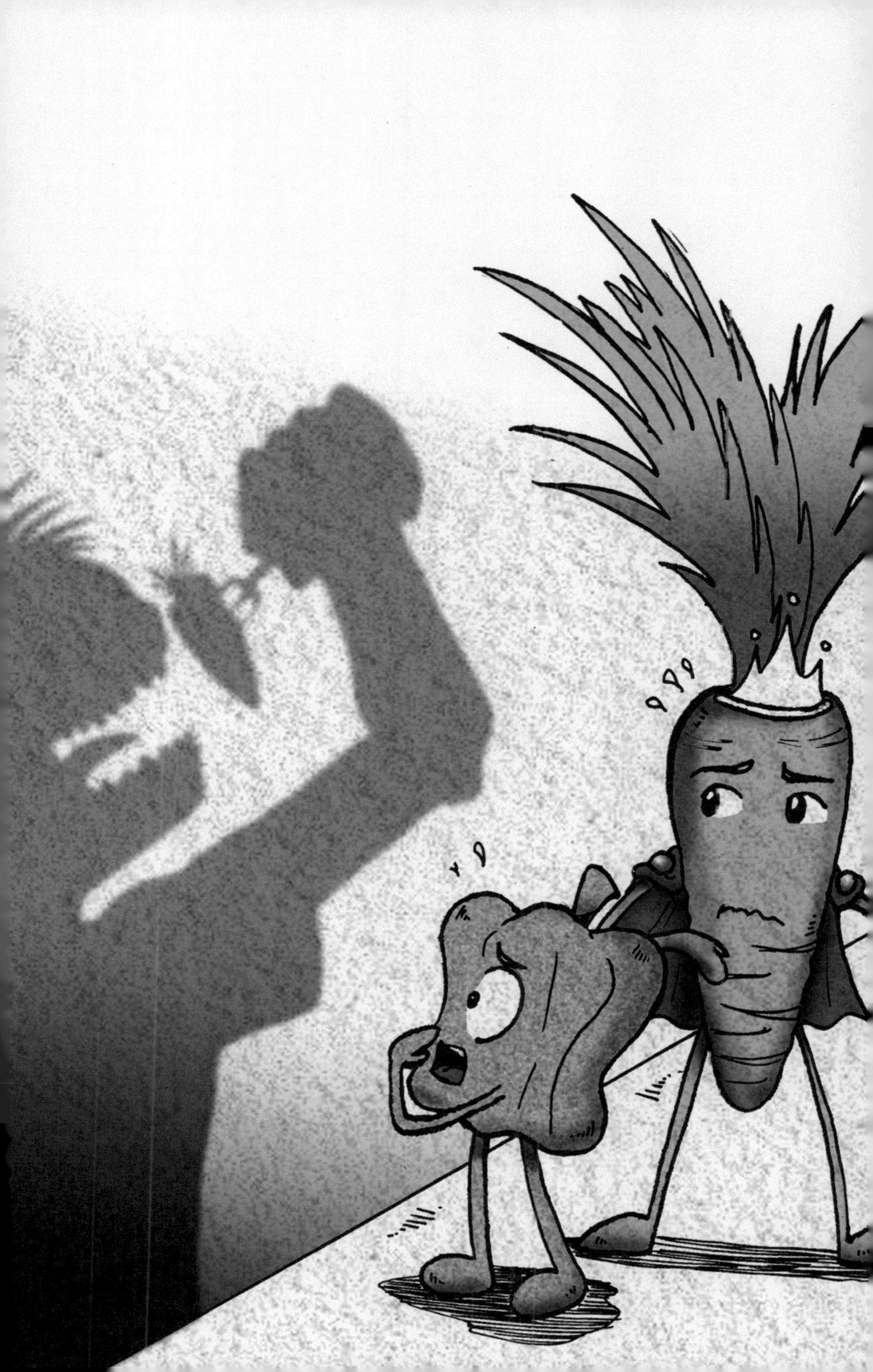

"I stagger and stare,
and groan like a zombie.
This last part is too hard,
please help me Mommy!"

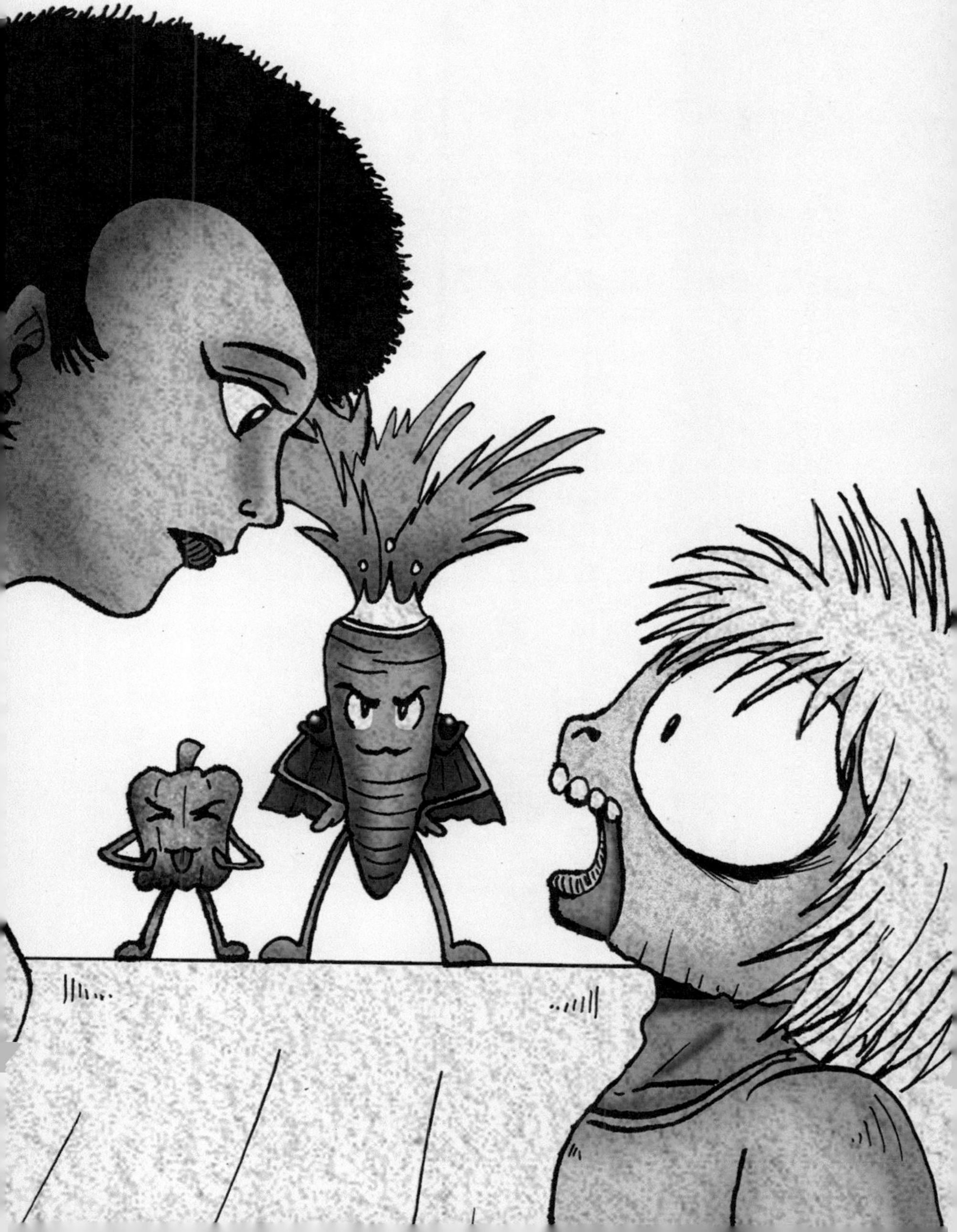

They smiled at young Tommy.
"Son, let us explain.
Zombies do not eat broccoli,
but we love broccoli brains!"

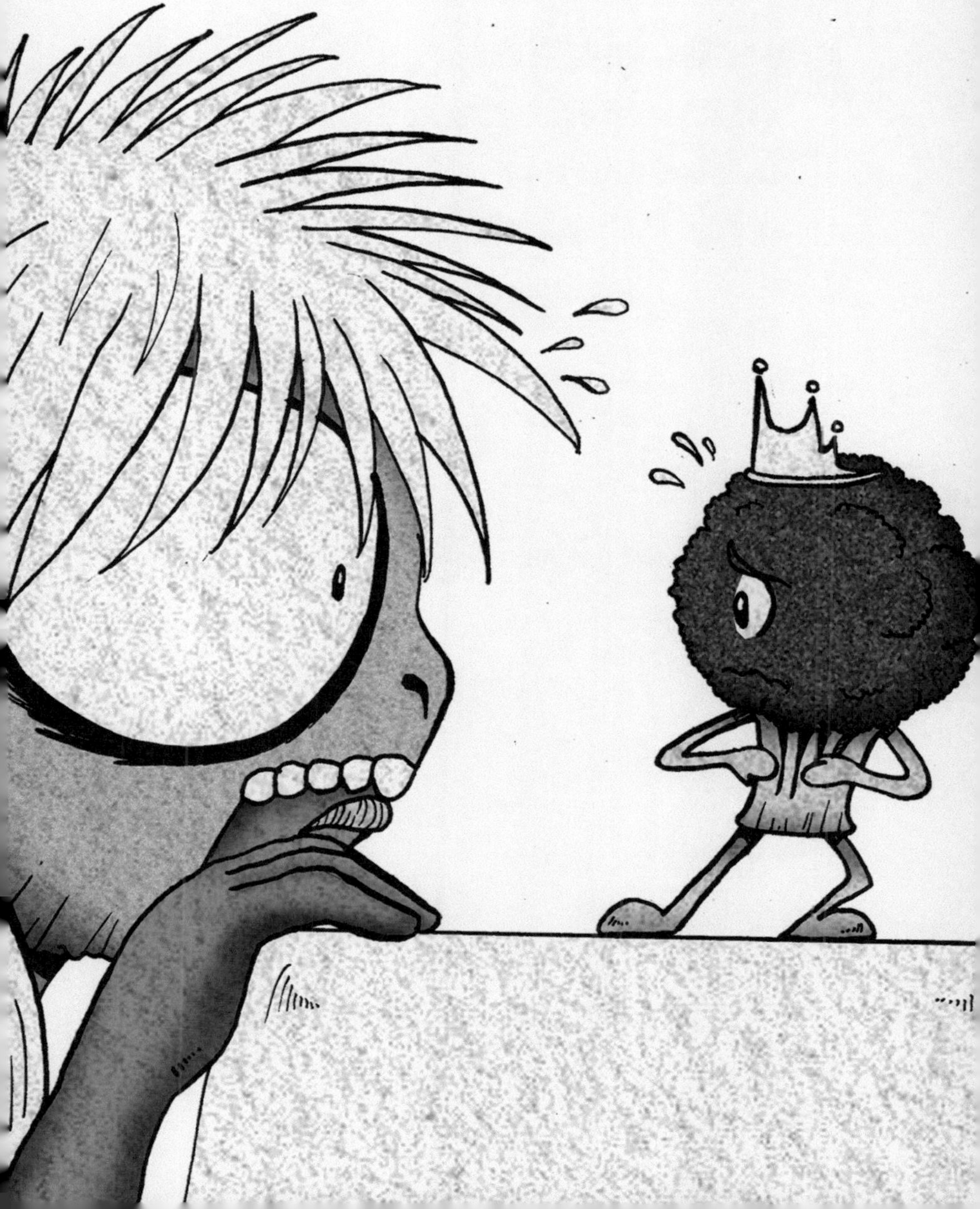

Well, carrots have brains,
And spinach does too!
But which is more scary,
the broccoli or you?"

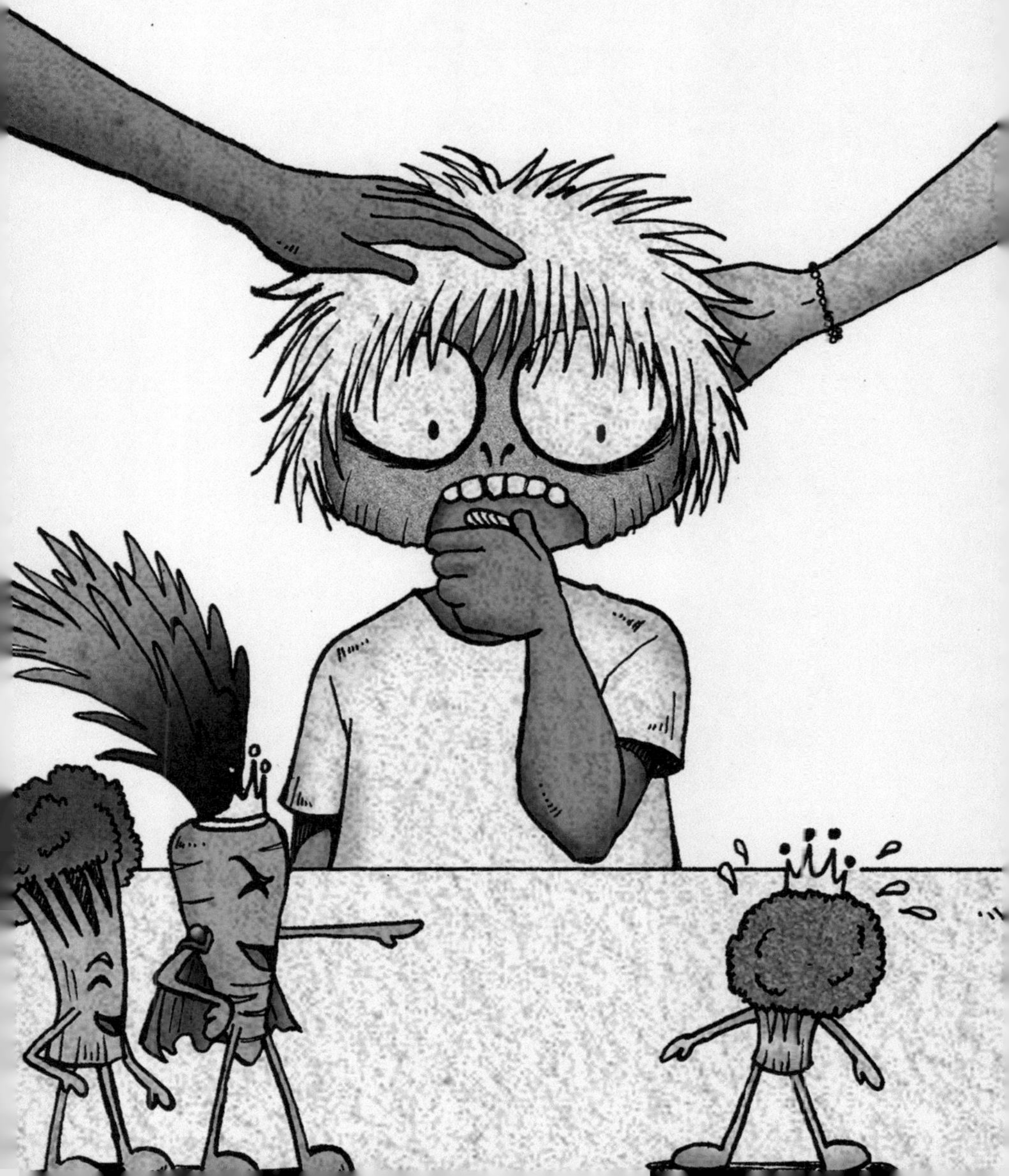

And so Tommy squinted.
His plate he reviewed.
He no longer saw vegetables,
only BRAIN FOOD.

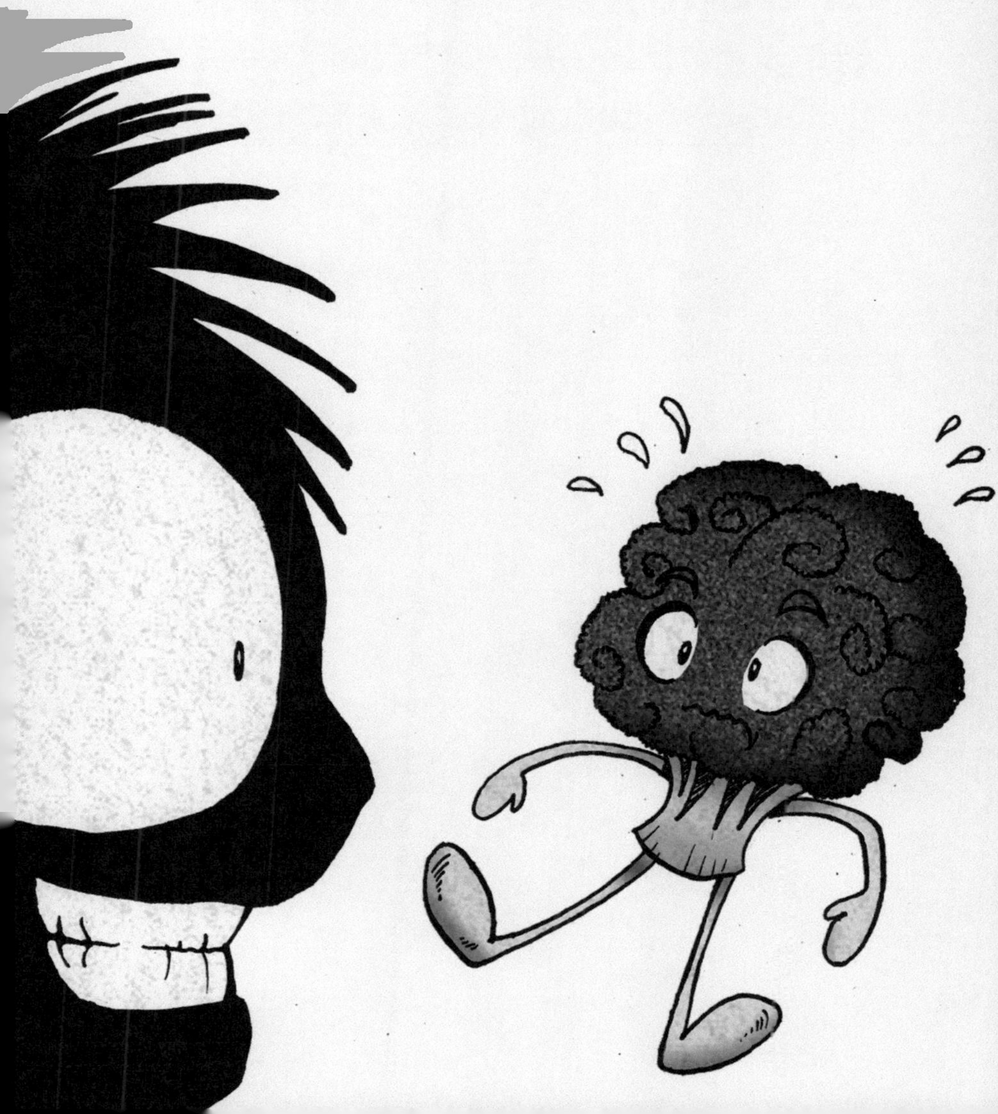

He poked with his fork,
he crunched and he chewed.
He swallowed and growled,
and finished his food.

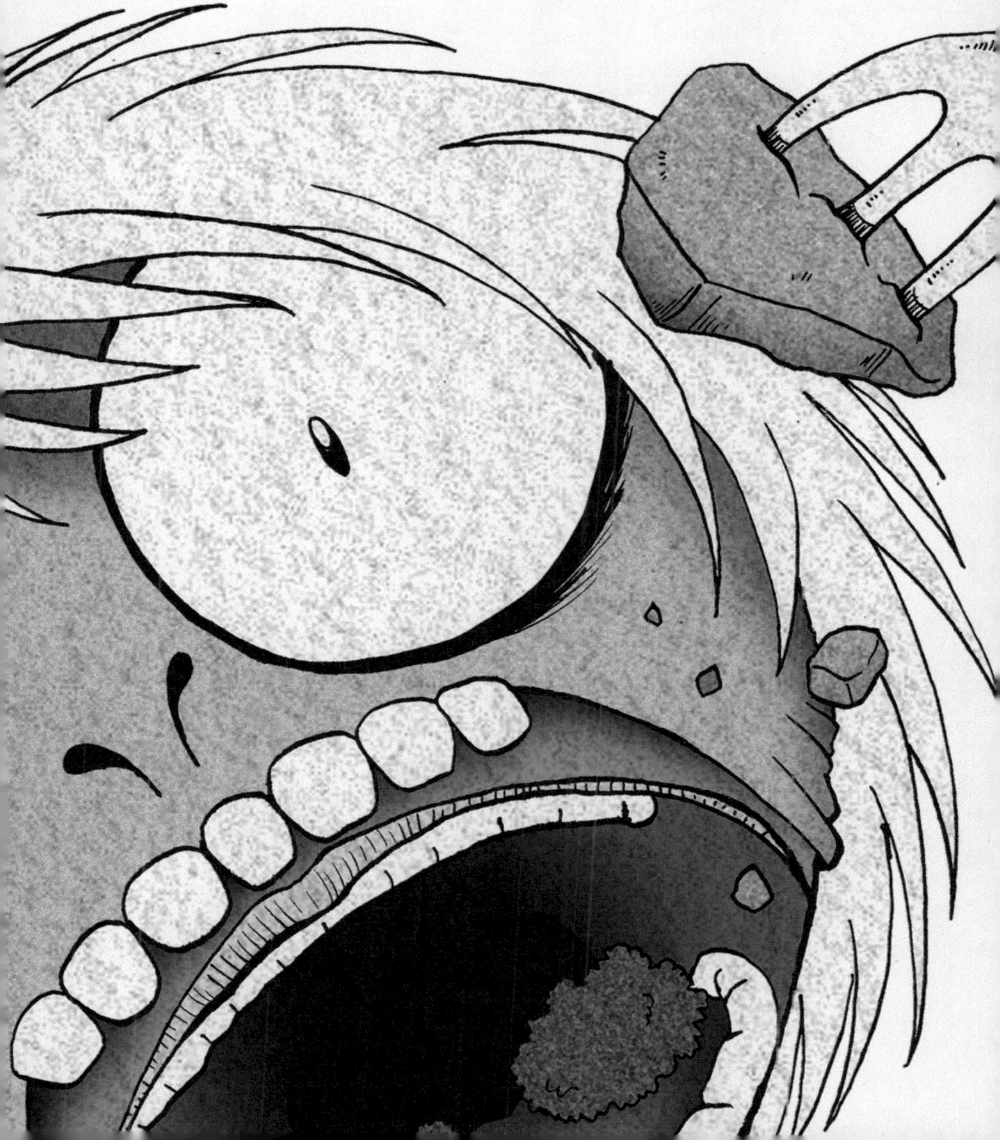

The next night there was cabbage,
and after that spinach.
Then carrots, then celery
and the bad taste diminished.

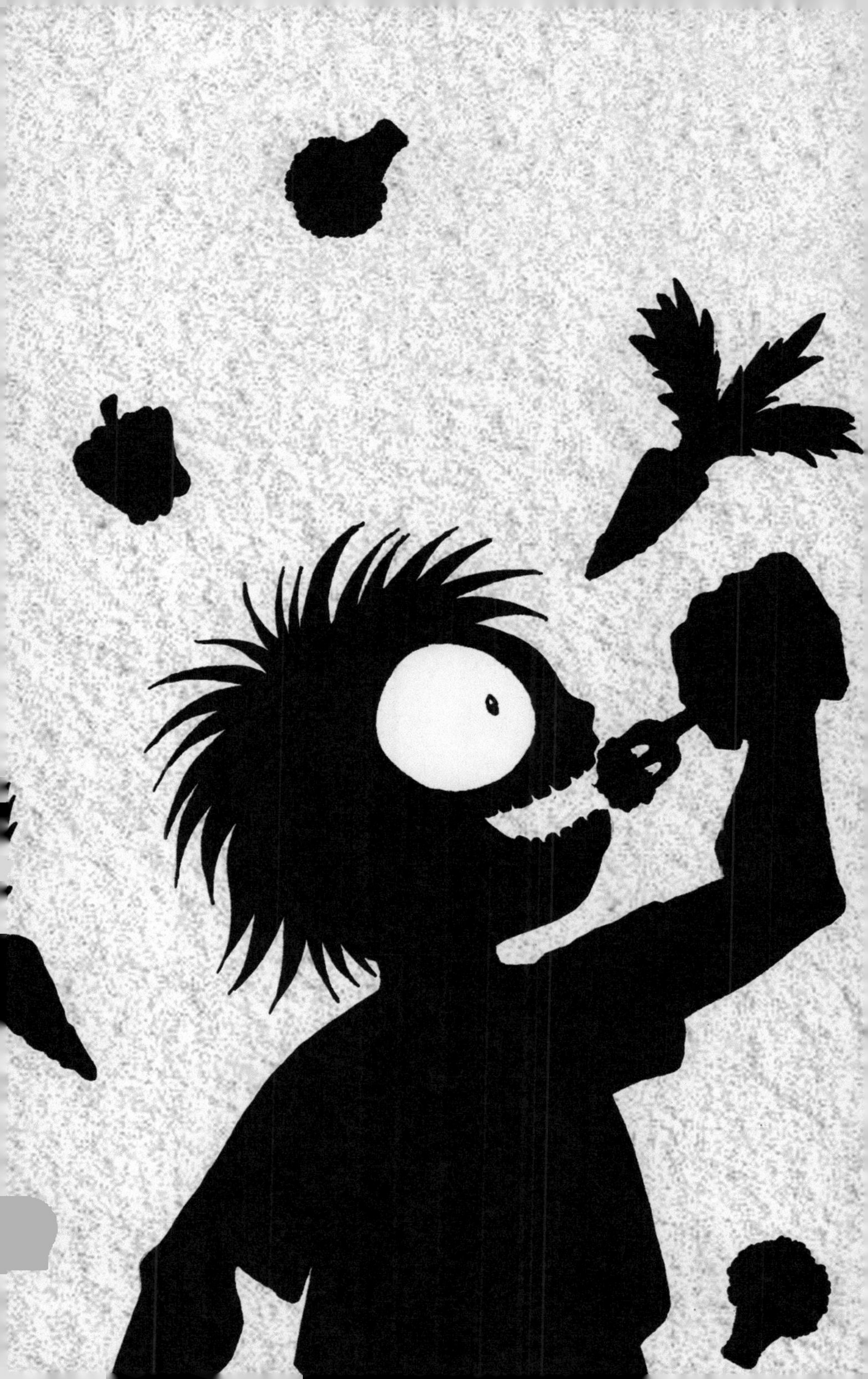

And in one short year
little Tommy had grown
to be stronger and smarter
than any zombie ever known.
No food was ever safe
(be it candy or cauliflower)
from Tommy the Zombie
and his new superpower.

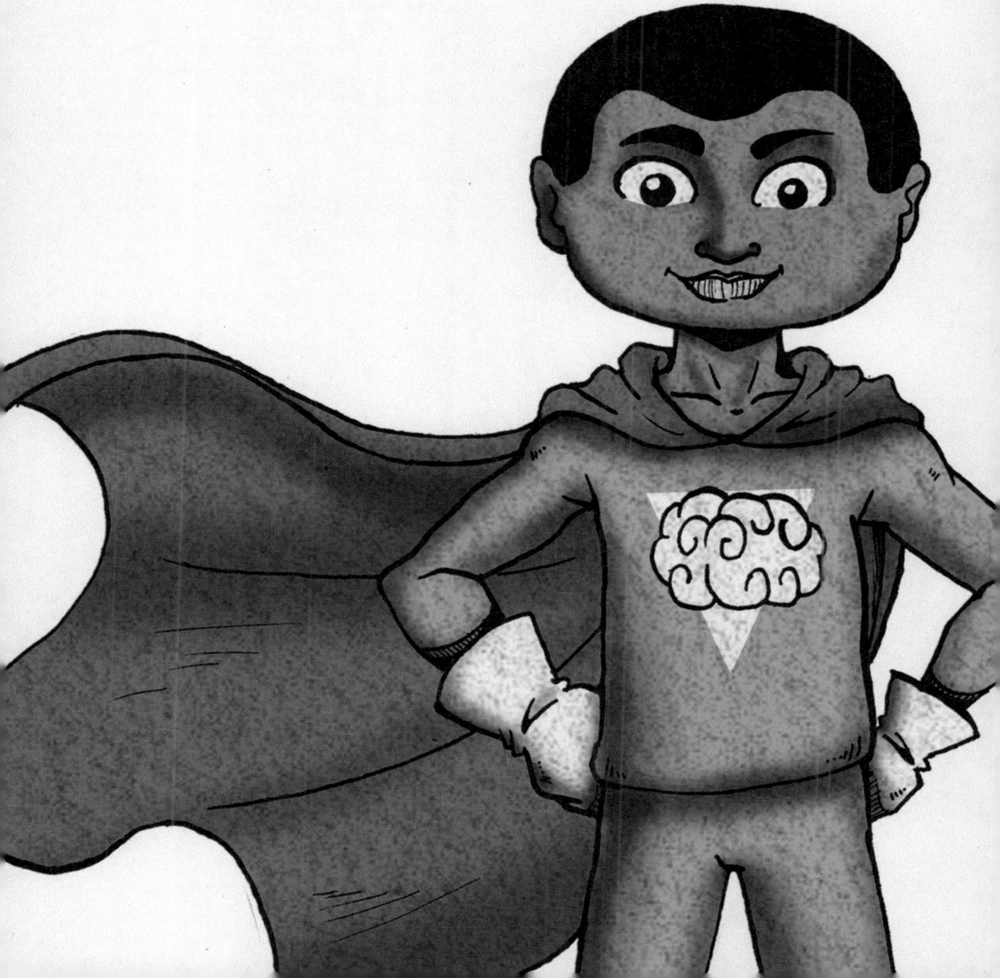

He could eat anything
Mommy or Daddy prepared
Green, yellow, or red
No vegetable spared.

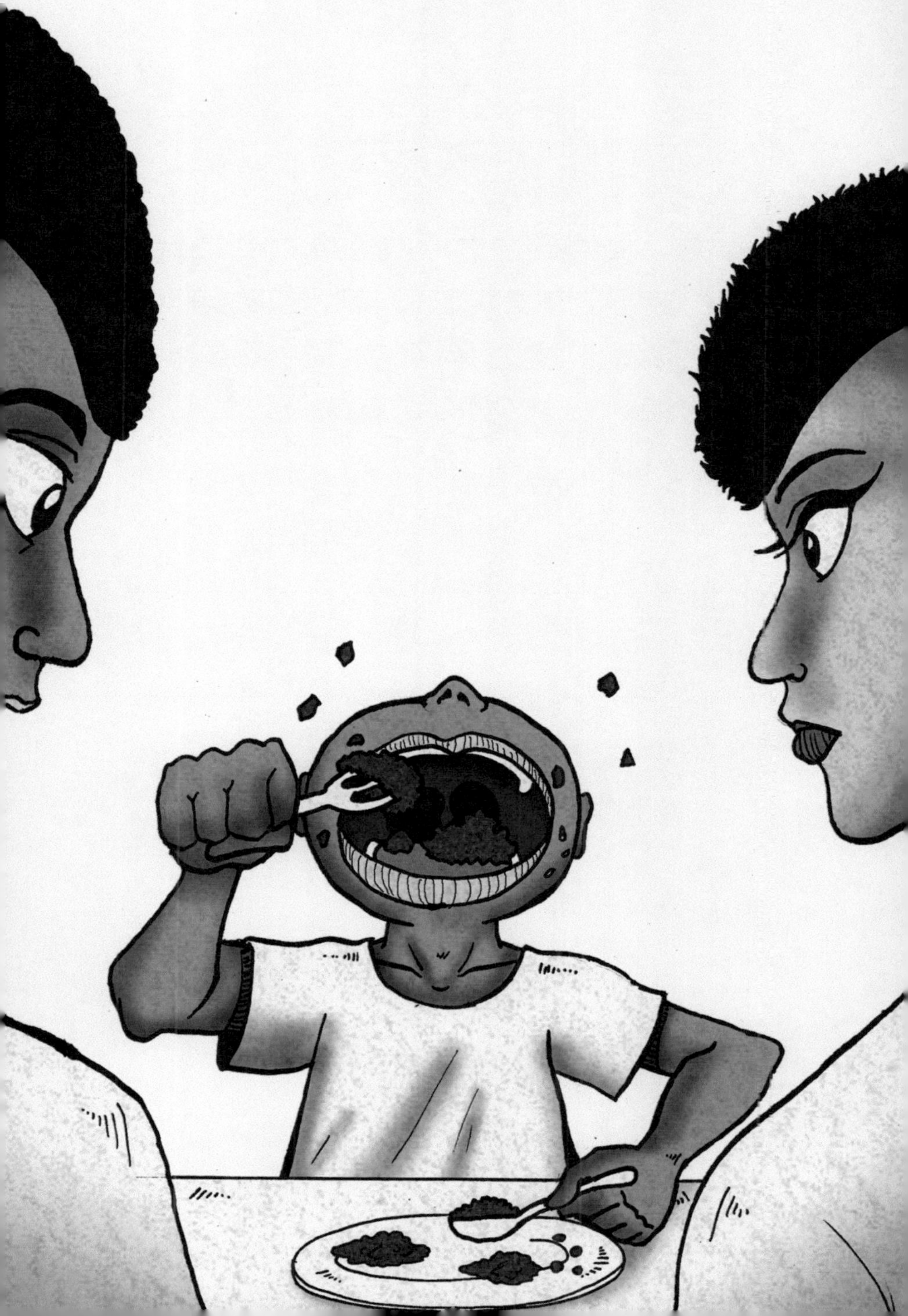

So if you're a fresh vegetable,
steamed, stewed, or strained
Beware the little zombie that could
devour your brains!

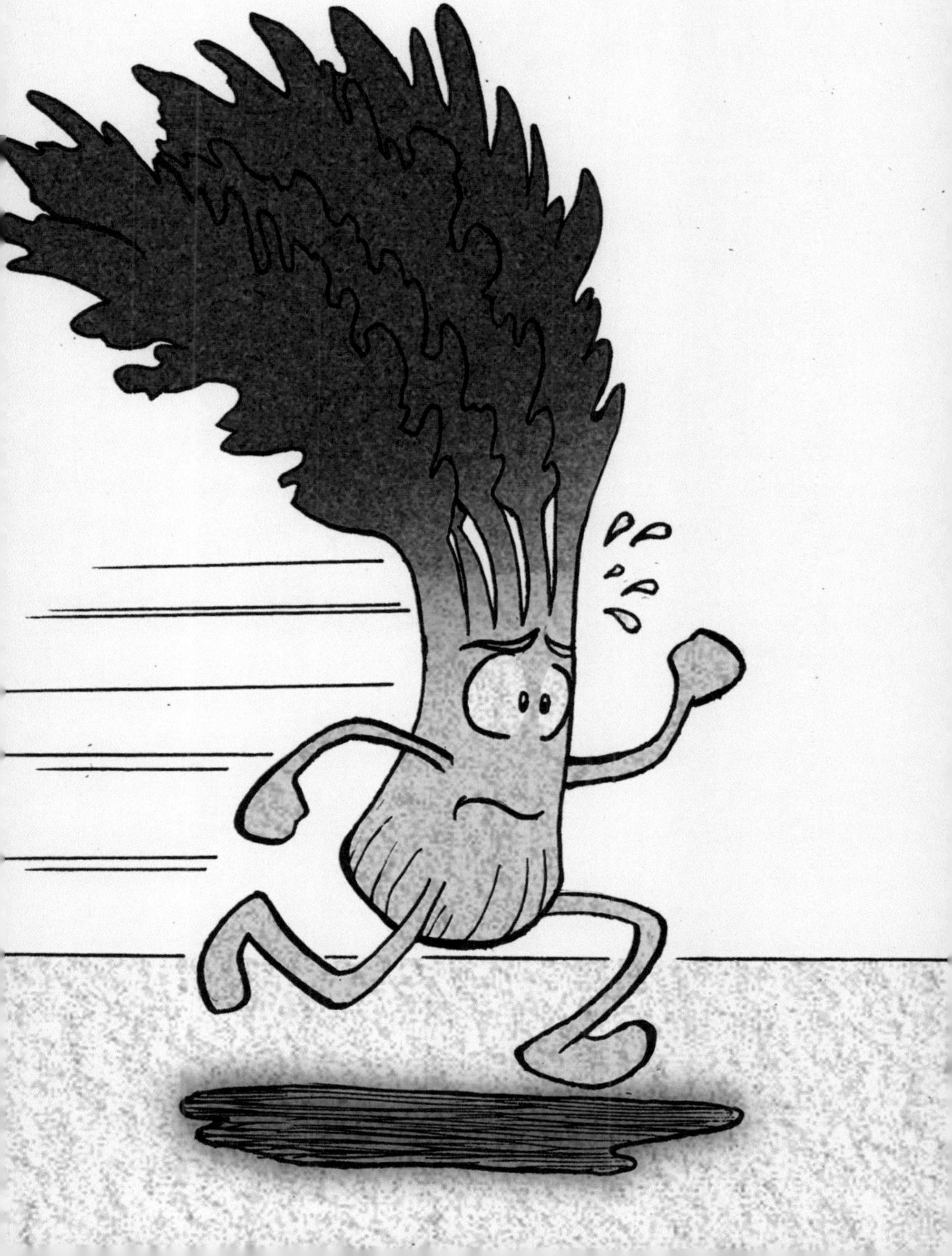

Made in the USA
Monee, IL
05 November 2026

67379786R00031